Multiple Sclerosis (MS)

Comprehensive Guide to Diagnosis, Treatment, Symptom Management, and Lifestyle Modifications for Living with Multiple Sclerosis

Graham Julian Oliver

Disclaimer

The information provided in this book is intended for general informational purposes only and should not be considered a substitute for professional medical advice, diagnosis, or treatment. The author and publisher make no representations or warranties about the completeness, reliability, or accuracy of the information contained herein. Always seek the advice of your physician or other qualified health provider with any questions you may have regarding a medical condition or treatment.

This book discusses various aspects of Multiple Sclerosis (MS), including diagnosis, treatment options, symptom management, and lifestyle modifications. However, individual experiences with MS can vary significantly, and the effectiveness of treatments and recommendations may differ based on individual circumstances. Therefore, it is essential to consult with a healthcare professional before making any changes to your treatment or lifestyle.

Furthermore, the author and publisher do not endorse any individual, product, website, organization, or other names mentioned in this book. Any references are included solely for informational purposes. The use of any products or services mentioned is at your own risk, and the author and publisher are not liable for any adverse effects or consequences resulting from the use of the information provided in this book.

By reading this book, you acknowledge that you have read, understood, and agreed to this disclaimer.

About This Book

The book *Multiple Sclerosis (MS): Comprehensive Guide to Diagnosis, Treatment, Symptom Management, and Lifestyle Modifications for Living with Multiple Sclerosis* serves as an essential resource for anyone seeking to understand and manage the complexities of living with MS. It begins by demystifying the condition, offering clear definitions of how MS affects the central nervous system and providing a comprehensive breakdown of the different types of MS, such as Relapsing-Remitting and Primary-Progressive. This foundational knowledge is critical for patients and caregivers alike, as it highlights the importance of early diagnosis and management, which can significantly impact the trajectory of the disease.

Diagnosis and treatment are thoroughly explored, covering the vital diagnostic tools, such as MRI and spinal taps, which neurologists use to identify and assess the progression of MS. The book emphasizes the importance of a multidisciplinary approach to care, which integrates the expertise of various healthcare professionals to tailor a personalized treatment plan. With detailed insights into disease-modifying therapies and symptom management medications, the guide offers practical knowledge that empowers patients to make informed decisions about their healthcare.

A significant focus is placed on understanding the disease process of MS, from the immune system's role to how the condition causes inflammation and nerve damage. The unpredictable nature of relapses and remissions is explained, along with how these fluctuations impact various bodily functions. This section also touches on factors that exacerbate MS symptoms, such as heat and stress, and provides an in-depth exploration of the invisible symptoms like fatigue and mood changes. These details ensure readers gain a holistic understanding of how MS manifests and progresses.

For those navigating a new diagnosis, the book offers practical advice on the steps involved in confirming MS, including the use of the McDonald criteria, and the challenges of diagnosis, particularly in the early stages.

It also addresses the emotional aspect of receiving a diagnosis, providing guidance on the next steps and debunking common myths surrounding the condition.

Treatment options and symptom management are a key focus, with extensive coverage of disease-modifying therapies and the pros and cons of different treatment approaches. The book outlines how to manage the most common symptoms, including fatigue, mobility issues, and cognitive challenges, and provides a balanced approach to combining medication with lifestyle modifications. The integration of non-drug approaches like exercise and mindfulness techniques adds a layer of support for patients seeking a more comprehensive strategy for symptom relief.

Living with MS requires daily life adjustments, and this guide delivers practical advice on managing energy, work environments, and mobility aids. It emphasizes the importance of maintaining flexibility in daily routines and offers solutions for managing memory issues, temperature sensitivity, and financial challenges. With tips on home modifications and planning for symptom flares, the book equips patients to navigate life with MS in a practical and sustainable way.

In the realm of nutrition, the book provides valuable insights into how diet can influence MS symptoms, particularly the role of anti-inflammatory diets and supplements like Omega-3s. It stresses the importance of maintaining a healthy weight and discusses how gut health and hydration can impact overall well-being. With special attention to how steroid treatments can affect weight and the potential benefits of working with a dietitian, the book underscores the role of nutrition in a holistic MS care plan.

Exercise and physical therapy are also vital components of MS management, and this guide highlights the benefits of regular activity, focusing on exercises tailored to improve mobility, reduce fatigue, and maintain strength. With practical suggestions on how to modify routines based on individual abilities, the book empowers readers to stay active and maintain their physical health despite the challenges posed by MS.

Emotional and mental health are equally important, and the book offers guidance on coping with the emotional impact of an MS diagnosis, including strategies for managing anxiety, depression, and mood swings. It stresses the value of psychological support, support groups, and mindfulness techniques, helping patients to build resilience and create a robust support network. This section ensures readers understand the psychological toll MS can take and provides practical strategies for emotional well-being.

Common concerns and detailed FAQs address pressing questions, such as the life expectancy of individuals with MS, the possibility of pregnancy, and concerns around mobility and independence. This section provides clear, fact-based answers to frequently asked questions, offering reassurance and clarity for those seeking to understand their long-term outlook.

Finally, the book emphasizes long-term management and lifestyle modifications, guiding readers on the importance of regular follow-up with neurologists, adapting to changing abilities, and maintaining a positive outlook. It discusses financial planning, staying updated with research, and developing a care plan with family and caregivers. The importance of preventive measures, such as avoiding secondary conditions and maintaining a healthy lifestyle, is underscored, providing a comprehensive roadmap for managing life with MS effectively over the long term.

In sum, this book is an indispensable resource for anyone navigating the complexities of MS, offering guidance that spans from diagnosis to long-term lifestyle adjustments, helping individuals manage the disease with knowledge, confidence, and hope.

Table of Contents

Introduction:

Definition of Multiple Sclerosis and How It Affects the Central Nervous System

Multiple Sclerosis (MS) is a chronic autoimmune disorder that targets the central nervous system (CNS), including the brain and spinal cord. It occurs when the immune system mistakenly attacks the protective covering of nerve fibers (myelin), causing communication problems between the brain and the rest of the body. Over time, this damage can lead to deterioration of the nerves themselves, resulting in physical and cognitive disability.

The CNS damage caused by MS disrupts the ability of nerves to transmit signals, which leads to a wide range of symptoms. These symptoms may vary significantly from one person to another, depending on the location and extent of the nerve damage. In severe cases, the condition can lead to paralysis, vision loss, and difficulties with coordination.

Types of MS: Relapsing-Remitting, Primary-Progressive, Secondary-Progressive, and Clinically Isolated Syndrome

Relapsing-Remitting MS (RRMS) is the most common form, characterized by flare-ups (relapses) followed by periods of partial or full recovery (remissions). Primary-Progressive MS (PPMS) is marked by a gradual worsening of symptoms without distinct relapses or remissions. Secondary-Progressive MS (SPMS) begins as RRMS but transitions into a progressive form where symptoms steadily worsen.

Clinically Isolated Syndrome (CIS) refers to a single episode of MS-like symptoms that last at least 24 hours. If additional episodes occur or MRI shows evidence of brain lesions, a diagnosis of MS may be confirmed. Early identification of these types is key to determining treatment strategies.

Early Warning Signs and Symptoms of MS

Early signs of MS can be subtle but include fatigue, vision problems (such as blurred or double vision), and numbness or tingling in the limbs. Muscle weakness, coordination difficulties, and balance problems may also be among the first symptoms noticed. Symptoms often appear between the ages of 20 and 40.

The unpredictable nature of these symptoms can make it challenging to detect MS in its early stages. Because the signs may be temporary or mistaken for other conditions, it is important to consult a healthcare professional when experiencing persistent or unusual neurological issues.

Prevalence and Risk Factors (Age, Gender, Genetics, Environmental Factors)

MS affects approximately 2.8 million people worldwide. It is more common in women than men, with a ratio of about 3:1. The onset of MS typically occurs between the ages of 20 and 40, but it can affect people of any age. Those with a family history of MS are at a slightly higher risk, suggesting a genetic component.

Environmental factors, such as living in regions farther from the equator, are linked to an increased risk of developing MS. This may be due to lower vitamin D levels, as sunlight exposure is believed to play a protective role. Smoking and certain viral infections, such as the Epstein-Barr virus, have also been identified as risk factors.

Importance of Early Diagnosis and Proactive Management

Early diagnosis of MS is crucial for managing the disease effectively. The sooner MS is diagnosed, the sooner treatment can begin, which can help delay the progression of the disease and reduce the severity of symptoms. Diagnosis typically involves MRI scans, spinal fluid analysis, and neurological exams to assess the extent of CNS damage.

Proactive management includes starting disease-modifying therapies (DMTs) to slow disease progression, addressing symptoms through medications and therapies, and making lifestyle adjustments. Early intervention can significantly improve quality of life by minimizing disability and preserving physical and cognitive function.

The Basics of MS Diagnosis and Treatment

Common Diagnostic Tools (MRI, Spinal Tap, Evoked Potentials)

Diagnosing multiple sclerosis (MS) often starts with imaging tests like Magnetic Resonance Imaging (MRI). An MRI scan detects lesions or damage in the brain and spinal cord caused by MS, making it one of the most reliable diagnostic tools. Alongside MRI, doctors may recommend a spinal tap (lumbar puncture) to check for abnormalities in cerebrospinal fluid. The presence of specific proteins can help confirm an MS diagnosis. Evoked potentials are another test that measures the electrical activity in response to stimuli, revealing nerve pathway damage that might not be visible on an MRI.

To undergo these tests, patients typically visit a hospital or diagnostic center. The MRI is non-invasive and requires the patient to lie still inside a large machine, while a spinal tap involves extracting fluid from the lower back under local anesthesia. Evoked potentials may involve attaching electrodes to the scalp or body. Together, these tools give neurologists a clear view of nervous system damage, helping them to diagnose MS more accurately.

The Role of Neurologists in MS Diagnosis and Treatment Planning

Neurologists play a crucial role in diagnosing and managing multiple sclerosis. They assess symptoms, order diagnostic tests, and analyze results to make a diagnosis. Once MS is confirmed, the neurologist develops a personalized treatment plan that addresses the patient's unique needs. They monitor disease progression, adjust medications as necessary, and provide guidance on managing symptoms and preventing relapses.

In practice, patients work closely with their neurologist during regular check-ups. The neurologist reviews test results, discusses treatment options, and explains the risks and benefits of each approach. As MS is a chronic condition, patients rely on their neurologist to modify the treatment plan over time, ensuring that it remains effective and adaptive to any changes in their condition.

Treatment Goals: Reducing Symptoms, Preventing Relapses, and Slowing Disease Progression

The primary goals in MS treatment are to reduce symptoms, prevent relapses, and slow the progression of the disease. Managing symptoms like fatigue, muscle weakness, and difficulty walking can improve quality of life. Preventing relapses, or flare-ups of new symptoms, is another key objective, as relapses can lead to permanent damage to the nervous system. Lastly, slowing the progression of MS helps minimize long-term disability and protect overall neurological function.

Achieving these goals requires a combination of medication, lifestyle changes, and ongoing care. Medications can reduce the frequency and severity of relapses, while physical therapy and lifestyle modifications help maintain mobility and energy. Regular check-ins with a neurologist ensure the treatment plan is working as intended and adjustments can be made when necessary.

Available Therapies (Disease-Modifying Therapies, Symptom Management Drugs)

Disease-modifying therapies (DMTs) are the cornerstone of MS treatment. These medications help slow disease progression and reduce the frequency of relapses. Some common DMTs include interferons, glatiramer acetate, and newer oral medications like dimethyl fumarate. These therapies are administered either through injection or orally and are tailored to the individual's needs and the severity of their MS.

In addition to DMTs, symptom management drugs address specific issues such as muscle spasms, bladder problems, or depression. Medications like baclofen or tizanidine are prescribed for muscle spasticity, while antidepressants may be used to manage mood changes. Together, these therapies work to maintain a higher quality of life and keep the symptoms of MS under control.

The Importance of a Multidisciplinary Approach to MS Care (Physicians, Therapists, Psychologists)

Managing MS often requires a team of specialists working together in a multidisciplinary approach. This includes neurologists, physical therapists, occupational therapists, and psychologists. Neurologists focus on diagnosing and treating the medical aspects of MS, while therapists help patients maintain physical function, manage fatigue, and adapt to any mobility challenges. Psychologists provide emotional support, helping patients cope with the mental health challenges that may arise due to chronic illness.

In practice, patients benefit from coordinated care where each specialist contributes to the overall management plan. For example, a physical therapist might design exercises to improve balance, while a psychologist helps patients deal with stress or anxiety. Regular communication among the care team ensures that all aspects of a patient's health are addressed comprehensively, improving outcomes and overall well-being.

CHAPTER 1:

Understanding the Disease Process of MS

Overview of How MS Affects the Immune System and Central Nervous System

Multiple Sclerosis (MS) occurs when the immune system mistakenly attacks the central nervous system (CNS), targeting the protective myelin sheath that surrounds nerve fibers. This process, called demyelination, leads to disrupted communication between the brain and body. As the immune system causes inflammation, it results in the formation of lesions (damaged areas) on the brain and spinal cord.

This disruption can cause a wide range of symptoms depending on the areas affected, such as movement issues or sensory disturbances. Over time, repeated attacks on the CNS can lead to permanent nerve damage, impacting overall function and quality of life for individuals with MS.

What Happens During a Relapse: Inflammation, Demyelination, and Nerve Damage

During an MS relapse (or flare-up), the immune system becomes highly active, leading to inflammation in the CNS. This inflammation damages the myelin sheath, leaving nerves exposed, which interrupts the electrical signals that travel through the nerves. This process is called demyelization and causes symptoms such as numbness, weakness, and vision problems.

If the inflammation persists, the nerve fibers themselves can become damaged, leading to more permanent effects. After the relapse subsides, some recovery may occur as inflammation decreases, but nerve damage can sometimes be irreversible, leading to lasting impairments.

The Difference Between Active and Inactive Lesions on MRI Scans

On MRI scans, active MS lesions indicate areas where new inflammation and demyelization are happening. These appear as bright spots and signal that the immune system is actively attacking the CNS. Active lesions often correlate with recent or ongoing symptoms.

Inactive lesions, on the other hand, are older areas of damage where inflammation has subsided. These appear darker on MRI scans and represent scar tissue left behind from previous attacks. Monitoring the development of both active and inactive lesions helps doctors assess disease progression.

Types of MS and Their Progression Patterns

There are four main types of MS: relapsing-remitting MS (RRMS), secondary-progressive MS (SPMS), primary-progressive MS (PPMS), and progressive-relapsing MS (PRMS). RRMS is the most common form, marked by periods of relapses followed by remission. SPMS occurs when RRMS transitions into a steadily worsening condition.

PPMS involve continuous disease progression without clear relapses, while PRMS is a rare type with both progression and occasional relapses. Each type follows its own unique progression, and individuals may experience varying degrees of disability over time.

Symptoms: Sensory Problems, Motor Issues, and Cognitive Impairment

MS can cause a variety of symptoms, often starting with sensory disturbances such as numbness, tingling, or vision problems. These occur because of the disrupted communication between the brain and affected nerves. Over time, motor issues like muscle weakness, spasticity, and impaired coordination can develop, making daily activities challenging.

Cognitive impairments, including memory loss, difficulty concentrating, and slowed thinking, can also arise. These symptoms often fluctuate and vary in intensity depending on the progression of the disease and the areas of the CNS affected by lesions.

How MS Lesions Impact Different Body Functions

MS lesions can develop in different parts of the brain and spinal cord, leading to a range of functional problems. Lesions in the optic nerves can cause vision issues, while lesions in the motor cortex can affect movement and coordination. Lesions in the brainstem or cerebellum may lead to balance problems and difficulty speaking or swallowing.

The location and size of the lesions determine the severity and type of symptoms experienced. Some individuals may experience only mild issues, while others face more severe impairments depending on the extent of nerve damage caused by the lesions.

The Role of Remyelination and Recovery between Relapses

After an MS relapse, the body attempts to repair the damage by replacing the lost myelin, a process called remyelination. In some cases, this can restore nerve function to a degree, allowing individuals to experience symptom relief during remission. However, remyelination is often incomplete, especially with repeated attacks, which can lead to long-term damage.

Between relapses, some recovery may occur, but the extent of healing varies from person to person. Effective management through medication and lifestyle changes can help reduce relapses and support better recovery between flare-ups.

Factors That Can Exacerbate MS Symptoms (Heat, Stress, Infections)

Certain factors can make MS symptoms worse or trigger a relapse. Heat is a common trigger, as higher temperatures can temporarily worsen symptoms like fatigue or muscle weakness, a phenomenon known as Uhthoff's phenomenon. Infections, even minor ones like colds, can also trigger relapses by over activating the immune system.

Stress plays a significant role in exacerbating MS symptoms, as it can weaken the body's ability to cope and cause flare-ups. Managing these factors through temperature control, stress reduction, and infection prevention is crucial for those living with MS.

How MS Is Different from Other Neurological Conditions

MS is an autoimmune disorder specifically targeting the CNS, which sets it apart from other neurological conditions. Unlike conditions like Parkinson's disease, which primarily affects movement, MS involves multiple areas of the CNS and presents with a wide range of sensory, motor, and cognitive symptoms.

Furthermore, MS is characterized by the formation of lesions in the brain and spinal cord due to immune system attacks, a feature not seen in many other neurological disorders. This makes MS unpredictable and variable in its presentation and progression.

Understanding the Invisible Symptoms of MS (Fatigue, Pain, Mood Changes)

MS is often called an "invisible illness" because many symptoms, such as fatigue, pain, and mood changes, aren't outwardly visible but significantly affect a person's quality of life. Fatigue is one of the most common and disabling symptoms, often unrelated to physical activity and challenging to manage.

Chronic pain, such as neuropathic pain from damaged nerves, is another common invisible symptom. Additionally, mood changes, including depression and anxiety, are frequent in people with MS due to both the physical impact of the disease and the psychological toll of managing a chronic illness.

MS Progression: From Benign to Severe Forms

MS can progress in various ways, with some individuals experiencing a benign form characterized by few symptoms and long periods of remission. However, others may have a more severe progression, where symptoms worsen over time, and periods of remission become shorter or disappear.

The severity of MS progression depends on several factors, including the frequency of relapses, the number of lesions, and the extent of nerve damage. Early intervention and treatment are crucial to slowing down progression and maintaining function as long as possible.

How Relapsing-Remitting MS Can Transition into Secondary-Progressive MS

In many cases, relapsing-remitting MS (RRMS) can transition into secondary-progressive MS (SPMS) after several years. During this transition, the pattern of distinct relapses followed by remission shifts to a more constant progression of symptoms without recovery between attacks.

This change can be gradual, and individuals may notice a steady worsening of symptoms, even in the absence of new relapses. Early and aggressive treatment of RRMS can help delay or potentially prevent the transition to SPMS.

The Unpredictability of MS and Its Long-Term Outlook

MS is notoriously unpredictable, with no two individuals experiencing the disease in the same way. Symptoms can come and go, progress slowly or rapidly, and affect various parts of the body. This uncertainty can make long-term planning and management challenging for individuals with MS.

While there is no cure for MS, advancements in treatments, including disease-modifying therapies, offer hope for slowing progression and managing symptoms.

Regular monitoring, lifestyle changes, and treatment adjustments help individuals navigate the unpredictability and improve their long-term outlook.

CHAPTER 2:

Diagnosis of Multiple Sclerosis

Early Signs That May Prompt an MS Evaluation

Early signs of multiple sclerosis (MS) may include unexplained fatigue, numbness, tingling, muscle weakness, or vision problems such as blurred or double vision. These symptoms can be subtle and mistaken for other conditions, but if they persist or worse, they may prompt a medical evaluation. People often notice episodes of imbalance, dizziness, or cognitive difficulties, which can vary from person to person.

If you experience these symptoms, it's essential to consult a doctor who can evaluate whether further tests for MS are necessary. Early detection allows for more effective management of the disease, helping to slow progression and improve quality of life.

Steps Involved in Ruling Out Other Conditions

Before diagnosing MS, doctors must rule out other conditions with similar symptoms. The process begins with a thorough physical exam and medical history review. Conditions such as lupus, Lyme disease, or vitamin deficiencies can mimic MS symptoms, so doctors will test for these first.

Additional tests, such as MRI scans, spinal fluid analysis, and blood work, are often conducted to exclude these alternative diagnoses. Once other conditions are ruled out, doctors will proceed with tests that focus on identifying MS-specific signs.

The Role of Medical History and Symptom Tracking

Medical history plays a crucial role in diagnosing MS. Patients are encouraged to track symptoms such as muscle weakness, balance issues, or vision problems over time. The doctor will ask about the onset, duration, and severity of symptoms to identify patterns that might suggest MS.

Symptom tracking is vital, as MS symptoms often come and go, making it challenging to diagnose. A detailed history helps doctors understand if these episodes are typical of MS relapses and remissions, aiding in diagnosis.

How MRI Imaging Identifies Lesions on the Brain and Spine

Magnetic Resonance Imaging (MRI) is one of the primary tools used to diagnose MS. MRI scans can reveal lesions or areas of damage on the brain and spinal cord, which indicate inflammation caused by MS. These lesions show up as bright spots on the MRI images, helping doctors pinpoint areas where nerve damage has occurred.

Doctors may order an MRI if MS is suspected based on symptoms. The presence of lesions, particularly in areas common for MS, supports the diagnosis and helps monitor disease progression over time.

Spinal Fluid Analysis and What It Reveals About Inflammation

A spinal tap (lumbar puncture) may be done to analyze cerebrospinal fluid (CSF) for signs of inflammation. In MS, the immune system attacks the central nervous system, which can cause proteins and antibodies to accumulate in the spinal fluid.

These markers help confirm MS by revealing the presence of oligoclonal bands, which indicate abnormal immune activity in the brain and spinal cord. The test can also help rule out other infections or conditions that could cause similar symptoms.

Evoked Potential Tests to Measure Nerve Responses

Evoked potential tests are used to measure the electrical activity of the brain in response to stimuli, such as visual or sensory input. These tests detect abnormalities in the speed or strength of nerve signals, which can be slowed by damage to the myelin sheath—a hallmark of MS.

The test is non-invasive and involves placing electrodes on the scalp. It helps detect silent lesions that might not cause immediate symptoms but still indicate nerve damage consistent with MS.

Blood Tests Used to Rule Out Other Autoimmune Diseases

Although there is no blood test to diagnose MS directly, blood tests are essential in ruling out other conditions that can mimic MS symptoms. Doctors may check for autoimmune diseases like lupus or Sjogren's syndrome, as well as infections such as HIV or Lyme disease.

These tests help narrow down the diagnosis by excluding other possible causes of neurological symptoms, ensuring that doctors focus on MS-specific evaluations.

When and Why a Neurologist Will Suggest Additional Testing

A neurologist may suggest further testing if the initial results are inconclusive or if the symptoms don't fully match MS criteria. Additional testing might include repeat MRIs, more in-depth spinal fluid analysis, or evoked potential tests to gather more evidence.

Neurologists aim to make a clear diagnosis while ensuring other conditions are ruled out. This cautious approach helps avoid misdiagnosis and ensures patients receive appropriate treatment for their specific condition.

How a Diagnosis Is Confirmed Through the McDonald Criteria

The McDonald criteria are the standard for diagnosing MS, combining clinical symptoms, MRI findings, and spinal fluid analysis to confirm a diagnosis. For MS to be confirmed, there must be evidence of damage in at least two separate areas of the central nervous system (CNS) at different points in time.

This approach ensures a precise diagnosis, as the criteria require proof of multiple attacks on the CNS over time, making it a reliable method for identifying MS.

Challenges in Diagnosing MS, Especially in the Early Stages

Diagnosing MS early can be difficult due to the variability of symptoms. MS symptoms often mimic other conditions, and initial episodes may be mild or intermittent. Because MS can take years to fully manifest, it can be hard for doctors to confirm without a clear pattern of neurological episodes.

MRI and other diagnostic tools help, but sometimes lesions are not immediately visible, complicating early diagnosis. For this reason, doctors often adopt a "wait and see" approach in the early stages of symptom presentation.

The Importance of Getting a Second Opinion When Diagnosis Is Unclear

When an MS diagnosis is unclear, seeking a second opinion is essential. Another neurologist might interpret test results differently or recommend additional tests to provide more clarity. Misdiagnosis is possible with MS, especially in the early stages, so confirming the diagnosis ensures the right treatment plan.

A second opinion can offer peace of mind and may also present new treatment or management options, helping patients move forward with confidence.

Emotional Responses to an MS Diagnosis and Next Steps

Receiving an MS diagnosis can be emotionally overwhelming. Many patients experience fear, confusion, or anxiety about what the future holds. It's important to seek support from healthcare providers, family, and MS support groups during this time.

Once diagnosed, the next step is to create a treatment plan with your doctor, which may involve medication, physical therapy, and lifestyle modifications. Early intervention can help manage symptoms and slow the progression of the disease.

Common Myths About MS Diagnosis

One common myth about MS is that the diagnosis is always immediate or clear-cut. In reality, MS can be difficult to diagnose, and the process may take time, especially in the early stages. Another misconception is that all MS patients will experience severe disability, though many people with MS live active, fulfilling lives with proper treatment.

Understanding these myths helps set realistic expectations and encourages proactive symptom management and communication with healthcare providers.

CHAPTER 3:

Treatment Options and Symptom Management

Disease-modifying therapies (DMTs) and their role in slowing MS progression

Disease-modifying therapies (DMTs) are critical in managing multiple sclerosis (MS), as they help reduce the frequency of relapses and slow the progression of disability. DMTs work by targeting the immune system to prevent further damage to the central nervous system, protecting the brain and spinal cord from inflammation. Starting a DMT early in the course of MS can improve long-term outcomes.

Choosing the right DMT depends on the type of MS, disease activity, and personal health factors. Neurologists will work with patients to identify the best therapy based on effectiveness, side effects, and individual preferences. Regular monitoring is essential to assess the efficacy and adjust the treatment as necessary.

Key differences between first-line and second-line DMTs

First-line DMTs are typically prescribed at the onset of MS and are known for having fewer side effects while still offering effective treatment. These include options like interferons and glatiramer acetate, which are often more tolerable for long-term use. They are generally prescribed for patients with less aggressive forms of MS.

Second-line DMTs are used when the disease is more active or when first-line therapies fail. These treatments, such as natalizumab or alemtuzumab, are more potent but come with higher risks of serious side effects, including infections or autoimmune conditions. Neurologists may recommend second-line options for those with rapidly progressing MS.

The pros and cons of oral vs. inject able treatments

Oral DMTs offer convenience since they don't require injections, making them more appealing for many MS patients. Examples include fingolimod and dimethyl fumarate. However, oral treatments may carry risks such as liver toxicity or gastrointestinal issues, and regular blood tests are often required for monitoring.

Injectable treatments, such as interferons or glatiramer acetate, are well-established and come with fewer systemic side effects. While injections can be inconvenient and may cause local skin reactions, they are generally considered safe and effective for long-term use.

Managing relapses with corticosteroids

Corticosteroids, such as methylprednisolone, are commonly used to manage MS relapses by reducing inflammation in the brain and spinal cord. These medications are typically administered in high doses over a few days to accelerate recovery from severe symptoms, such as vision loss or mobility issues.

While corticosteroids can be effective in controlling relapses, they are not used long-term due to potential side effects like weight gain, insomnia, or bone thinning. They are a short-term solution and should be part of a broader treatment plan involving DMTs and symptom management strategies.

Treating fatigue, the most common symptom of MS

Fatigue in MS is often overwhelming and can significantly impact daily life. Managing fatigue involves a combination of lifestyle changes, energy conservation techniques, and medications like amantadine or modafinil. Patients are encouraged to balance activities with rest periods to avoid overexertion.

Simple changes like staying hydrated, improving sleep hygiene, and maintaining a healthy diet can help alleviate fatigue. Exercise, despite feeling counterintuitive, can boost energy levels and improve overall well-being, reducing the intensity of MS-related fatigue.

Pain management: medications and alternative therapies

MS-related pain can vary from nerve pain to musculoskeletal discomfort. Medications like gabapentin or pregabalin are often prescribed to manage neuropathic pain, while nonsteroidal anti-inflammatory drugs (NSAIDs) may help with muscle and joint pain.

Alternative therapies such as acupuncture, massage, and mindfulness meditation can complement medication by addressing pain holistically. Physical therapy may also help in reducing muscle tension and improving mobility, contributing to pain relief.

Addressing mobility issues: physiotherapy, assistive devices

Mobility issues are common in MS due to muscle weakness, spasticity, or balance problems. Physiotherapy is a key treatment, offering exercises that improve strength, balance, and coordination. Therapists work with patients to develop customized programs based on their specific mobility challenges.

Assistive devices like canes, walkers, or orthotic supports can help patients maintain independence and safety. Occupational therapists may also recommend home modifications to reduce the risk of falls, ensuring that daily activities remain manageable.

Cognitive rehabilitation for memory and focus difficulties

Cognitive rehabilitation involves structured activities designed to improve memory, attention, and problem-solving skills in MS patients. Therapists use exercises that train the brain to compensate for deficits, helping patients develop strategies to manage cognitive changes effectively.

Simple tools like calendars, reminder apps, and task lists can aid in daily memory and organizational challenges. Consistent mental exercises, combined with lifestyle changes like adequate sleep and reduced stress, can improve focus and cognitive function over time.

Managing bladder and bowel symptoms

Bladder and bowel issues, such as urgency, incontinence, or constipation, are common in MS. Managing these symptoms involves behavioral techniques, such as timed bathroom visits and pelvic floor exercises. In some cases, medications like anticholinergics may help control bladder spasms.

Dietary adjustments, such as increasing fiber intake or staying hydrated, are essential for managing bowel problems. In more severe cases, catheters or laxatives may be required under medical supervision to ensure comfort and health.

Medications for spasticity and muscle stiffness

Muscle stiffness and spasticity can be debilitating for MS patients, affecting mobility and comfort. Baclofen or tizanidine are common medications prescribed to reduce muscle tightness. These medications help relax the muscles and make movement easier.

Physical therapy, stretching, and hydrotherapy can also play a significant role in managing spasticity. Regular exercise, particularly in warm water, can reduce muscle tension and improve flexibility without overstraining muscles.

Non-drug approaches for symptom relief (exercise, meditation, etc.)

Non-drug approaches like exercise and meditation are highly beneficial for MS patients. Regular physical activity, such as swimming or yoga, improves muscle strength, flexibility, and overall mood, helping to manage fatigue and mobility issues. Low-impact exercises are recommended to avoid straining muscles.

Mind-body practices like meditation, deep breathing, and mindfulness can alleviate stress, which is known to exacerbate MS symptoms. These techniques can also help manage pain, promote relaxation, and improve emotional well-being.

Combining medication with lifestyle changes for better symptom control

A comprehensive approach that combines medication with lifestyle changes is crucial for managing MS symptoms effectively. Medications like DMTs reduce disease activity, while complementary strategies such as regular exercise, a balanced diet, and stress management can improve overall quality of life.

Lifestyle changes, such as prioritizing sleep, staying hydrated, and engaging in social activities, can also enhance symptom control. Regular check-ups with a neurologist ensure that treatment plans are adapted to the patient's evolving needs.

The importance of ongoing monitoring and adjusting treatment plans

Ongoing monitoring of MS is essential to track disease progression and treatment efficacy. Regular MRI scans, blood tests, and neurological evaluations help doctors assess how well DMTs are working and detect any new or worsening symptoms. Adjustments to the treatment plan can then be made as needed.

Patients should report any changes in symptoms to their healthcare provider promptly. By maintaining open communication and staying proactive in their care, patients can ensure that their treatment remains effective in managing MS over the long term.

CHAPTER 4:

Living with MS: Daily Life Adjustments

How MS Affects Daily Routines and the Need for Flexibility

Living with Multiple Sclerosis (MS) requires flexibility in daily routines due to unpredictable symptoms like fatigue, muscle weakness, and cognitive changes. It's essential to prioritize tasks, break activities into manageable segments, and allow for rest breaks throughout the day. Staying adaptable helps maintain a balance between responsibilities and energy levels.

Flexibility also means being ready to adjust your day based on how you feel. If fatigue hits hard, shifting priorities or rescheduling activities can help. Using planners, alarms, and reminders allows you to stay organized without feeling overwhelmed, making it easier to manage your day when symptoms fluctuate.

Energy Conservation Techniques to Manage Fatigue

MS-related fatigue can be one of the most challenging symptoms to manage. Energy conservation techniques, like the "4 P's" (Prioritize, Plan, Pace, and Position), help in managing tasks more efficiently. Prioritizing tasks ensures that essential activities are completed first. Planning the day ahead helps avoid overexertion.

Pacing yourself is crucial—takes regular breaks and spread tasks throughout the day to avoid burning out. Positioning, or sitting while performing activities like cooking, reduces physical strain. These techniques prevent energy depletion and create a manageable daily routine.

Adapting Work Environments for MS-Friendly Productivity

Adapting your work environment to suit MS can improve comfort and productivity. Simple changes, like ergonomic chairs, voice-activated software, or a flexible schedule, can significantly reduce fatigue. Creating a clutter-free, organized space and using task management tools can help with memory issues and brain fog.

It's also helpful to communicate with your employer about any needed adjustments, such as working from home or modifying workloads. Many employers are willing to accommodate with small but effective changes, helping you maintain both productivity and health.

Managing Temperature Sensitivity and Heat Intolerance

Heat sensitivity, common in people with MS, can worsen symptoms like fatigue and muscle weakness. Staying in a cool environment is key to managing this. Cooling aids like vests, fans, and cold packs can help keep body temperature regulated during warmer months or while exercising.

Avoiding hot showers or prolonged sun exposure also reduces the risk of exacerbating symptoms. Keeping rooms well-ventilated and wearing light, breathable clothing can also make a significant difference in comfort and daily function.

Mobility Aids: When and How to Use Them

Mobility aids, such as canes, walkers, or wheelchairs, can be vital tools for maintaining independence with MS. It's important to assess your mobility needs with a healthcare professional, who can recommend the right aid for your specific situation. Canes may be used to help balance, while wheelchairs might be necessary for longer distances or periods of weakness.

Using these tools when needed can prevent falls, reduce fatigue, and help you move around safely. Incorporating aids into daily life shouldn't be viewed as a setback but rather a proactive step in maintaining mobility and independence.

The Role of Occupational Therapy in Simplifying Tasks

Occupational therapy (OT) can offer practical solutions for everyday challenges caused by MS. An occupational therapist can assess how MS affects your routine tasks and provide strategies or adaptive tools to make them easier. For instance, using jar openers, grab bars, or reaching aids can reduce strain.

OT also includes energy conservation techniques, helping you find ways to modify activities to be less physically or mentally draining. Whether it's at work or home, OT equips you with tools and methods that allow you to perform daily tasks more comfortably and efficiently.

Strategies for Managing Memory Issues and Brain Fog

Cognitive symptoms like memory loss and brain fog are common in MS. To manage these, keeping a structured routine and using reminders, checklists, and apps can help you stay on track. Breaking tasks into smaller steps and avoiding multitasking can also make it easier to focus.

Practicing cognitive exercises or using brain-training apps may improve memory and focus over time. Setting realistic goals and taking breaks when needed allows you to manage cognitive symptoms without feeling overwhelmed.

Practical Tips for Navigating MS-Related Vision Problems

Vision issues, such as blurred vision or double vision, can occur in MS. When experiencing these problems, it's helpful to adjust your environment, such as increasing font sizes on devices or using contrasting colors in your living space to improve visibility. Using magnifying glasses or audio books can also assist in daily tasks.

If light sensitivity is an issue, wearing sunglasses or using filters on screens can provide relief. Working with an eye specialist is also important, as they can suggest treatments or strategies like prism glasses to help manage vision challenges.

Communicating Your Needs and Limitations to Family and Colleagues

Effectively communicating your needs to family and colleagues is essential in managing MS. Being clear about your limitations, whether it's needing breaks, avoiding certain activities, or asking for specific accommodations, helps others understand your situation. Open conversations help set expectations and avoid misunderstandings.

You can also use written communication tools, such as emails or task lists, to ensure clarity in professional settings. Regular check-ins with colleagues or family members provide opportunities to adjust as your symptoms change, helping to maintain good relationships and support networks.

Financial Planning and Managing Medical Costs Related to MS

Managing the financial burden of MS involves careful planning. It's crucial to explore insurance options, including coverage for medications, therapies, and medical equipment. Financial advisors specializing in healthcare can offer strategies for managing these expenses, such as opening health savings accounts or exploring government assistance programs.

Budgeting for out-of-pocket costs, travel for medical appointments, and potential future care should be factored in as well. By organizing finances early, you can focus on managing your health without the added stress of financial instability.

Making Home Modifications for Ease and Accessibility

Modifying your home can greatly enhance comfort and accessibility with MS. Installing grab bars in bathrooms, using non-slip mats, or widening doorways for wheelchair access are practical steps to improve mobility. Adjusting lighting, adding ramps, and rearranging furniture can reduce tripping hazards and make everyday tasks easier.

It's also helpful to have key items, like medications or frequently used objects, in accessible locations. Home modifications can be as simple as organizing your space or more extensive, depending on your individual needs, but they make life more manageable and safe.

Planning for Unpredictable Symptom Flares

Symptom flares are an unpredictable aspect of MS, so planning ahead is essential. Keep an "emergency flare plan," including rest periods, quick access to medications, and adjustments in your schedule. Informing your family or caregivers of what to expect during flares can reduce stress and help them provide better support.

It's also useful to avoid triggers like stress or extreme temperatures, as these can bring on a flare. Having a support system and a flexible mindset can make symptom flares more manageable without disrupting your entire routine.

Balancing Independence with Accepting Help When Needed

Maintaining independence is important, but knowing when to ask for help can prevent unnecessary stress and exhaustion. Gradually accepting assistance, whether from family, friends, or professionals, can improve your quality of life. It might be as simple as letting someone run errands or help with physical tasks when you're feeling fatigued.

Balancing independence with help allows you to conserve energy for the activities that matter most to you. Developing a strong support network ensures that you have help when needed while still maintaining control over your daily life.

CHAPTER 5:

Nutrition and MS: Diet and Supplements

The Role of Nutrition in Managing MS Symptoms

Nutrition plays a crucial role in managing multiple sclerosis (MS) symptoms. A balanced diet can help improve energy levels, maintain immune function, and promote overall health. Focusing on whole foods, such as fruits, vegetables, lean proteins, and whole grains, can provide essential nutrients that support bodily functions. For beginners, it's helpful to keep a food diary to track what you eat and how it affects your symptoms, as individual responses to food can vary widely.

In addition to whole foods, incorporating specific nutrients may further aid in symptom management. For example, antioxidants found in colorful fruits and vegetables can help combat oxidative stress, which is believed to contribute to MS progression. Beginners should consider consulting with a healthcare professional to create a personalized nutrition plan tailored to their specific symptoms and health goals.

Anti-Inflammatory Diets: How They Help Reduce MS Flares

Anti-inflammatory diets focus on reducing inflammation in the body, which can help alleviate symptoms and decrease the frequency of MS flare-ups. These diets emphasize foods rich in omega-3 fatty acids, such as fatty fish, walnuts, and flaxseeds, alongside plenty of fruits, vegetables, whole grains, and healthy fats like olive oil. For those new to anti-inflammatory diets, meal planning can simplify the process; consider preparing meals in advance that include a variety of these beneficial foods.

To implement an anti-inflammatory diet, begin by gradually replacing processed and sugary foods with whole foods. Start by incorporating one anti-inflammatory meal per day and slowly increase this to include more throughout the week. Familiarizing yourself with recipes that feature these ingredients can also make it easier to stick to the diet and enjoy the flavors.

The Importance of Maintaining a Healthy Weight

Maintaining a healthy weight is essential for managing MS, as being overweight can exacerbate symptoms and increase the risk of other health issues. A practical approach to weight management includes regular physical activity, balanced nutrition, and mindful eating. Begin by setting realistic weight goals and incorporating daily activities that you enjoy, such as walking, swimming, or yoga, which can make exercise feel less daunting.

To manage your weight effectively, monitor your caloric intake and ensure you're consuming a balanced diet. Keeping a food diary can help identify eating patterns and areas for improvement. Consider portion control techniques, such as using smaller plates or measuring out servings, to help you stay on track with your goals without feeling deprived.

Omega-3s and Other Supplements That May Benefit MS

Omega-3 fatty acids have been shown to possess anti-inflammatory properties that may help alleviate MS symptoms. For beginners, incorporating omega-3-rich foods such as salmon, chia seeds, and walnuts into your diet is a great starting point. If dietary sources are insufficient, consider discussing supplementation with a healthcare provider to determine the appropriate dosage for your needs.

In addition to omega-3s, other supplements such as magnesium, B vitamins, and probiotics may benefit overall health and well-being. Beginners should research reputable supplement brands and consult with a healthcare professional before starting any new regimen to ensure it's safe and beneficial for their specific health conditions.

Foods to Avoid That May Exacerbate Symptoms

Certain foods may worsen MS symptoms, including those high in saturated fats, trans fats, and added sugars. For beginners, identifying and eliminating these foods can help reduce flare-ups and improve overall health. Start by reading food labels to recognize these ingredients, and focus on consuming whole, minimally processed foods whenever possible.

Additionally, some individuals may find that dairy or gluten aggravates their symptoms. Keep a food diary to track your symptoms in relation to specific foods and consider an elimination diet, under the guidance of a healthcare professional, to pinpoint potential triggers. Gradually reintroducing eliminated foods can help identify any adverse reactions.

The Role of Vitamin D in MS Management

Vitamin D plays a vital role in immune function and has been linked to MS management. Many people with MS have low levels of vitamin D, making it essential to monitor and possibly supplement this nutrient. For beginners, safe sun exposure, dietary sources such as fortified foods, fatty fish, and egg yolks, or vitamin D supplements can help increase levels. A simple blood test can determine your current vitamin D status, allowing for tailored supplementation.

Incorporating vitamin D into your routine can be straightforward; aim for regular sun exposure and consider fortified foods. If supplementation is necessary, consult with a healthcare provider to determine the appropriate dosage and to ensure it aligns with your overall health strategy. Tracking your vitamin D intake can also help in maintaining adequate levels.

Hydration: Why it's Crucial for MS Patients

Staying hydrated is essential for everyone, but it is particularly important for those with MS, as dehydration can lead to increased fatigue and worsen other symptoms. A practical approach to hydration is to aim for at least eight 8-ounce glasses of water a day, but individual needs may vary. Beginners can track their water intake with apps or by keeping a water bottle handy to remind themselves to drink throughout the day.

In addition to plain water, incorporating hydrating foods such as fruits and vegetables can also boost overall fluid intake. Consider adding slices of lemon, cucumber, or berries to your water for a refreshing flavor. Establishing a daily hydration routine, such as drinking a glass of water before meals or setting reminders, can help ensure you meet your hydration goals.

Managing Weight Gain from Steroid Treatments

Steroid treatments can lead to weight gain, making it essential for those with MS to develop strategies to manage this side effect. Begin by discussing weight management with your healthcare provider, who can help create a personalized plan that includes dietary adjustments and physical activity. Focusing on a balanced diet rich in fruits, vegetables, whole grains, and lean proteins can help mitigate weight gain while still providing necessary nutrients.

Incorporating regular physical activity can also counteract weight gain from steroids. Aim for at least 150 minutes of moderate exercise each week, incorporating both aerobic and strength-training activities. Finding enjoyable activities, such as group classes or outdoor walks, can make it easier to stay active and maintain a healthy weight.

How Gut Health May Affect MS and Autoimmune Diseases

Emerging research suggests that gut health plays a significant role in autoimmune diseases, including MS. A healthy gut microbiome can help modulate immune responses, potentially reducing MS symptoms. For beginners, focusing on a diet rich in fiber from fruits, vegetables, and whole grains can support gut health. Additionally, incorporating fermented foods like yogurt, kefir, and sauerkraut can introduce beneficial probiotics into the gut.

To further improve gut health, consider minimizing processed foods and added sugars that can negatively impact the microbiome. Tracking your dietary intake and symptoms can help identify which foods promote a healthier gut environment. Consulting with a healthcare provider can also provide tailored guidance on optimizing gut health for your individual needs.

Supplements That May Help with Fatigue and Overall Well-Being

Fatigue is a common symptom of MS, and certain supplements may help alleviate it while promoting overall well-being. B vitamins, especially B12, play a crucial role in energy production, so including foods rich in these vitamins or considering supplementation may be beneficial. For beginners, a balanced diet that includes whole grains, lean meats, and legumes can help provide these essential nutrients.

Other supplements, such as coenzyme Q10 and iron, may also support energy levels. Before starting any new supplement, it's essential to consult with a healthcare provider to ensure they're appropriate for your specific situation. Keeping a symptom journal can also help identify which supplements or dietary changes positively affect your energy levels.

Importance of a Balanced Diet in Managing Overall Health with MS

A balanced diet is vital for overall health and wellness, particularly for individuals living with MS. It provides essential nutrients that support the immune system, maintain energy levels, and improve overall quality of life. Beginners should focus on creating meals that include a variety of food groups, such as fruits, vegetables, whole grains, lean proteins, and healthy fats, ensuring they receive a wide array of nutrients.

Meal prepping can simplify maintaining a balanced diet, allowing you to plan and prepare nutritious meals in advance. Start with a weekly meal plan that includes diverse foods to keep meals interesting and satisfying. By making small changes, such as incorporating one new fruit or vegetable each week, you can gradually enhance your overall diet and health.

How to Work with a Dietitian to Customize a Nutrition Plan

Working with a registered dietitian can help you create a customized nutrition plan that aligns with your health goals and MS management. A dietitian can provide personalized guidance, taking into account your specific symptoms, dietary preferences, and lifestyle. For beginners, finding a dietitian who specializes in MS or autoimmune diseases can ensure that you receive targeted support.

To make the most of your sessions with a dietitian, come prepared with questions about your dietary habits, symptoms, and any concerns you may have. Collaborate on setting realistic goals and developing meal plans that are practical for your lifestyle. Regular follow-ups can help track progress and adjust the plan as needed to ensure ongoing support in managing your health.

Special Dietary Needs During Relapses and Recovery

During relapses and recovery from MS symptoms, special dietary considerations may be necessary to support the body's healing processes. Focus on nutrient-dense foods that promote immune function, such as fruits, vegetables, and lean proteins. During a relapse, it's important to listen to your body's needs and consider smaller, more frequent meals to maintain energy levels without overwhelming your system.

Consulting with a healthcare provider or dietitian can provide tailored guidance on dietary adjustments during these periods. They can help identify any specific nutrients you may need more of, such as protein or vitamins, and suggest easy-to-prepare meals that fit your changing energy levels and symptoms. Keeping a flexible approach to your diet can help you navigate these challenging times while prioritizing your health.

CHAPTER 6:

Exercise and Physical Therapy for MS

The Benefits of Regular Exercise for MS Patients

Regular exercise is crucial for individuals with Multiple Sclerosis (MS) as it helps to improve overall health and well-being. Engaging in physical activity can lead to enhanced mobility, reduced fatigue, and better emotional health. Studies have shown that those who maintain a consistent exercise routine often experience less severe symptoms and a higher quality of life. Additionally, exercise can help manage the physical limitations associated with MS, promoting independence and encouraging a more active lifestyle.

To reap the benefits of exercise, it's essential to find enjoyable activities that fit into one's daily routine. Starting with small, manageable sessions can prevent overexertion and ensure consistency. Incorporating exercises like stretching, balance training, and cardiovascular activities can create a well-rounded program that addresses various symptoms of MS. It is advisable to consult with a healthcare provider or an MS specialist to create a tailored exercise plan that meets individual needs and abilities.

How Exercise Improves Mobility and Reduces Fatigue

Exercise significantly enhances mobility for MS patients by strengthening muscles and improving coordination. Regular activity can lead to better balance, allowing individuals to perform daily tasks with greater ease. Additionally, aerobic exercises increase cardiovascular fitness, which helps boost energy levels and reduce feelings of fatigue. This is particularly important for those with MS, as fatigue is one of the most common and debilitating symptoms.

By consistently incorporating exercise into their routine, individuals can experience a gradual improvement in their stamina and endurance. This can be achieved through simple activities such as walking, swimming, or cycling. These low-impact exercises can be adapted to suit varying levels of mobility, making it easier for individuals to remain active without excessive strain.

Types of Exercises Best Suited for People with MS

Various types of exercises are beneficial for those living with MS, including yoga, swimming, and walking. Yoga promotes flexibility, balance, and relaxation, making it an excellent choice for managing MS symptoms. Swimming is also highly effective, as the buoyancy of water reduces strain on the joints while providing a full-body workout. Walking, whether indoors or outdoors, can easily be adapted to different fitness levels and offers a great way to stay active.

In addition to these activities, incorporating light strength training can further enhance physical abilities. It's essential to choose exercises that are enjoyable and sustainable to ensure long-term adherence. Starting with 10 to 15 minutes a day and gradually increasing the duration can help build confidence and ability over time.

How to Modify Exercises Based on Individual Mobility Levels

Modifying exercises based on individual mobility levels is crucial for preventing injury and ensuring safety. People with MS should assess their capabilities and choose exercises that match their current strength and balance. For example, seated exercises or using a chair for support during standing exercises can help individuals who may struggle with balance. Additionally, lighter weights or resistance bands can be utilized to adjust the intensity of strength training.

It's also important to listen to one's body and make adjustments as needed. If a particular exercise causes discomfort, substituting it with a gentler option is advisable. Gradually increasing the complexity or intensity of workouts as strength improves can foster a sense of achievement and motivation.

The Role of Physical Therapy in Managing MS-Related Muscle Weakness

Physical therapy plays a vital role in managing muscle weakness associated with MS. A trained physical therapist can develop a personalized exercise program that focuses on strength building, flexibility, and endurance. Through targeted exercises, patients can improve muscle function and regain lost mobility, which is essential for daily activities. Physical therapists can also provide hands-on treatments that help alleviate pain and stiffness.

Incorporating physical therapy into a treatment plan can lead to significant improvements in quality of life. Patients often report feeling more empowered and capable of performing tasks they once found challenging. Regular sessions can ensure that exercises are performed correctly, preventing injury and maximizing benefits.

Stretching Exercises to Reduce Muscle Stiffness

Stretching exercises are essential for reducing muscle stiffness and maintaining flexibility in MS patients. Simple stretches can be performed daily to target tight areas and promote relaxation. Focusing on major muscle groups, such as the hamstrings, quadriceps, and back, can help alleviate discomfort and improve mobility. Stretching before and after workouts is particularly beneficial in preventing injuries and easing muscle tension.

Incorporating stretching into the daily routine can also foster mindfulness and relaxation, further enhancing emotional well-being. Many individuals find it helpful to use guided stretching videos or work with a physical therapist to ensure proper techniques are used. Maintaining a consistent stretching schedule can lead to long-term improvements in flexibility and comfort.

Using Resistance Training to Build Strength without Overexertion

Resistance training is a practical way for individuals with MS to build strength while minimizing the risk of overexertion. Utilizing resistance bands or light weights can provide sufficient resistance to strengthen muscles without excessive strain. Aiming for 2 to 3 sessions per week, focusing on major muscle groups, can yield significant benefits. It is essential to start with lower weights and gradually increase them as strength improves.

To maximize the effectiveness of resistance training, it's beneficial to incorporate exercises that mimic daily activities, making them functional. For instance, performing seated leg lifts or modified push-ups can enhance muscle strength while ensuring safety. Tracking progress and adjusting weights as needed will foster a sense of achievement and encourage continued participation.

Balance Exercises to Reduce the Risk of Falls

Balance exercises are crucial for reducing the risk of falls in individuals with MS, as instability can lead to serious injuries. Simple exercises such as standing on one leg, heel-to-toe walking, or using a balance board can help improve coordination and stability. It's essential to practice these exercises in a safe environment, ideally with a sturdy support surface nearby, to prevent accidents.

Incorporating balance training into a regular exercise routine can provide significant long-term benefits. Over time, improved balance will contribute to greater confidence in movement and allow individuals to engage more fully in daily activities. Regular practice of these exercises can help enhance overall physical resilience.

How to Avoid Overheating During Exercise

Avoiding overheating during exercise is particularly important for individuals with MS, as heat can exacerbate symptoms. To prevent overheating, it is advisable to exercise in cooler environments, wear breathable clothing, and stay well-hydrated before, during, and after physical activity. Taking breaks and resting when feeling overheated can also be beneficial in managing body temperature.

Utilizing techniques such as exercising during cooler parts of the day or engaging in water-based activities can help maintain a comfortable body temperature. Keeping a fan nearby or using cooling towels can further assist in regulating body heat. Being aware of one's body and recognizing the signs of overheating can empower individuals to adapt their routines effectively.

Finding a Safe and Effective Exercise Routine with an MS Specialist

Working with an MS specialist or a certified exercise physiologist can significantly enhance the effectiveness and safety of an exercise routine. These professionals can provide personalized guidance, ensuring that exercises are tailored to meet individual abilities and limitations. They can also help set realistic goals and track progress, which is crucial for maintaining motivation and accountability.

Finding a safe routine involves assessing personal preferences and physical capabilities. Together with the specialist, patients can explore different activities and modify them based on energy levels and overall health. Regular check-ins can help adjust the routine as necessary, ensuring continued benefits and improvements over time.

The Psychological Benefits of Staying Active with MS

Staying active offers numerous psychological benefits for individuals with MS, including reduced anxiety and improved mood. Engaging in regular exercise can promote the release of endorphins, which are known to enhance feelings of happiness and well-being. Additionally, participating in group activities can foster a sense of community and support, combating feelings of isolation often experienced by those with chronic conditions.

By setting and achieving fitness goals, individuals can experience a boost in self-esteem and confidence. Maintaining a routine of physical activity also provides a sense of control and purpose, helping to manage the emotional challenges associated with living with MS. It is essential to choose enjoyable activities that resonate personally to encourage long-term participation.

Developing a Flexible Routine to Accommodate Fluctuating Energy Levels

Creating a flexible exercise routine that accommodates fluctuating energy levels is essential for those living with MS. Individuals should prioritize activities that can be adjusted based on daily energy levels, allowing them to maintain consistency without overexertion. This might include short bursts of activity, such as 10-15 minute sessions, combined with rest periods to recharge.

Incorporating a variety of exercises can also keep routines interesting and adaptable. For example, mixing low-impact aerobic exercises, strength training, and stretching can provide a balanced approach that suits varying energy levels. Keeping a journal to track energy levels and activities can help identify patterns, making it easier to plan workouts that fit into daily life.

Tracking Progress and Adjusting Exercises Over Time

Tracking progress is vital for individuals with MS as it helps to monitor improvements and adjust exercise plans accordingly. Keeping a log of exercises performed, duration, and how one felt afterward can provide valuable insights into what works best. This can help in identifying strengths, areas for improvement, and exercises that may need modification.

Adjusting exercises over time based on progress is crucial for continued success. As strength, endurance, and confidence grow, increasing the intensity or duration of workouts can help maintain motivation and challenge the body. Regularly reviewing goals and celebrating achievements, no matter how small, can foster a positive mindset and encourage ongoing commitment to physical activity.

CHAPTER 7:

Emotional and Mental Health Support

Recognizing the Emotional Impact of an MS Diagnosis

Receiving a diagnosis of multiple sclerosis (MS) can be overwhelming and can trigger a range of emotional responses. Many individuals experience feelings of shock, confusion, and grief as they adjust to the reality of living with a chronic illness. It's essential to acknowledge these emotions rather than suppress them, as recognizing the emotional impact is the first step toward coping effectively. Understanding that these feelings are valid can help you start the process of acceptance and adaptation.

To navigate this emotional landscape, it's crucial to seek support from healthcare professionals who can provide guidance and resources. Connecting with mental health specialists who understand MS can help you develop coping strategies tailored to your unique situation. Engaging in open discussions about your feelings can also aid in reducing feelings of isolation and promote emotional healing.

Dealing with Anxiety, Depression, and Mood Swings

Anxiety and depression are common among individuals with MS due to the uncertainty of the disease and its symptoms. Recognizing the signs of anxiety—such as persistent worry or panic attacks—and depression—such as prolonged sadness or loss of interest in activities—is vital. If you experience these symptoms, consider reaching out to a healthcare provider for evaluation and support.

Managing these emotional challenges often involves a combination of therapy, medication, and lifestyle adjustments. Cognitive-behavioral therapy (CBT) can be effective in helping you reframe negative thoughts and develop healthier coping mechanisms. Additionally, medication may be prescribed to help stabilize mood and reduce anxiety, providing a more balanced emotional state.

The Importance of Counseling and Psychological Support

Counseling can play a critical role in helping individuals cope with the emotional challenges of MS. A trained mental health professional can provide a safe space to explore feelings, develop coping strategies, and gain insight into the emotional aspects of living with a chronic illness. Regular sessions can help you process emotions and provide tools to manage stress and anxiety.

It's essential to find a counselor who understands MS and its complexities. This specialized knowledge ensures that the support provided is relevant and empathetic to your experiences. Engaging in counseling can lead to improved mental health, greater self-awareness, and enhanced resilience in facing the challenges of MS.

Joining Support Groups to Connect with Others Living with MS

Joining a support group can be an invaluable resource for those living with MS. These groups offer a platform to connect with others who share similar experiences, fostering a sense of community and understanding. Sharing personal stories can help alleviate feelings of isolation, as members often find solace in knowing they are not alone in their struggles.

Support groups may meet in person or online, providing flexibility for participation. During these gatherings, individuals can share coping strategies, resources, and encouragement, all of which contribute to emotional well-being. Engaging with others who understand your journey can empower you to navigate the challenges of MS more effectively.

How MS Affects Self-Esteem and Body Image

MS can significantly impact self-esteem and body image, especially as symptoms change over time. Physical challenges, fatigue, and mobility issues can lead to feelings of inadequacy and frustration. It's important to recognize that these changes do not define your worth or abilities. Acknowledging your strengths and accomplishments can help rebuild a positive self-image.

Practical steps to improve self-esteem include engaging in activities that promote body positivity and celebrating personal achievements, no matter how small. Surrounding yourself with supportive friends and family who appreciate you for who you are—beyond your illness—can also enhance your self-image and reinforce a positive outlook on life.

Coping Strategies for MS-Related Cognitive Changes

Cognitive changes, such as memory lapses and difficulty concentrating, are common among those with MS. To cope with these challenges, consider implementing strategies that can help improve cognitive function. Techniques such as using planners, checklists, and reminders can aid in managing daily tasks and appointments effectively.

Additionally, engaging in cognitive exercises—like puzzles, memory games, or learning new skills—can help stimulate the brain and improve mental agility. Regular physical exercise and maintaining a balanced diet can also support overall brain health, contributing to better cognitive function and resilience against cognitive changes.

Mindfulness and Relaxation Techniques to Manage Stress

Mindfulness and relaxation techniques can be effective tools for managing stress associated with MS. Practicing mindfulness involves focusing on the present moment and accepting thoughts and feelings without judgment. Techniques such as meditation, deep breathing, and yoga can help you cultivate mindfulness, reducing anxiety and promoting emotional balance.

Incorporating these practices into your daily routine can lead to increased relaxation and improved overall well-being. Start with short sessions and gradually increase the duration as you become more comfortable. Establishing a consistent practice can create a sense of calm and improve your ability to cope with the stressors of living with MS.

Communicating Emotional Needs with Family and Friends

Open communication about your emotional needs is crucial for building strong support systems. Share your feelings with family and friends, letting them know how they can help you during difficult times. Being honest about your struggles fosters understanding and can lead to a deeper connection with loved ones.

Consider setting aside regular time for discussions about your emotional well-being. Encourage your support network to ask questions and express their feelings as well. This two-way communication can create an environment where everyone feels valued and understood, making it easier to address challenges as they arise.

Coping with the Uncertainty of Disease Progression

Living with MS often involves coping with uncertainty regarding disease progression and potential flare-ups.

To manage these feelings, focus on what you can control, such as maintaining a healthy lifestyle and adhering to treatment plans. Developing a routine can provide structure and help mitigate anxiety related to unpredictability.

Additionally, practicing acceptance can reduce the emotional burden of uncertainty. Engage in activities that bring you joy and fulfillment, helping to shift your focus away from worry. Support groups can also offer reassurance by allowing you to share experiences with others navigating similar challenges.

Strategies for Handling Social Isolation Due to MS

Social isolation is a common issue for individuals with MS, often exacerbated by mobility challenges and fatigue. To combat isolation, explore ways to maintain connections with friends and family, such as virtual meetups or phone calls. Regular communication can help you feel less alone and remind you of the support available to you.

Participating in local MS support groups or community activities can also provide opportunities for social interaction. Many organizations offer events tailored to individuals with MS, creating an inclusive environment for networking and friendship-building. Engaging with others who understand your experiences can alleviate feelings of isolation and enhance your emotional well-being.

The Role of Medication in Treating MS-Related Mood Disorders

Medications play a crucial role in managing mood disorders associated with MS, such as depression and anxiety. If you're experiencing significant emotional challenges, consult your healthcare provider about possible pharmacological interventions. They can evaluate your symptoms and recommend appropriate medications tailored to your specific needs.

It's essential to work closely with your healthcare team to monitor the effects of medication, as individual responses can vary. Regular follow-ups can help ensure that your treatment plan remains effective, providing you with the best possible support for managing mood-related issues.

Resilience Building: Staying Positive Amid Challenges

Building resilience is vital for navigating the ups and downs of living with MS. Start by identifying your strengths and focusing on positive aspects of your life. Setting achievable goals can help create a sense of purpose and accomplishment, reinforcing a positive mindset despite challenges.

Incorporating daily practices such as gratitude journaling or affirmations can further enhance resilience. Reflecting on what you're thankful for or affirming your strengths can shift your focus from difficulties to possibilities, promoting a healthier outlook on life and bolstering your ability to cope with MS-related challenges.

Creating a Support Network for Emotional Well-Being

Establishing a strong support network is key to managing the emotional aspects of living with MS. Reach out to friends, family, healthcare providers, and support groups to create a diverse network of support. Having various resources allows you to access different perspectives and forms of assistance, which can be invaluable during tough times.

Consider setting up regular check-ins with trusted friends or family members to discuss your feelings and experiences. This proactive approach fosters open communication and strengthens your support network, ensuring you have people to turn to when facing challenges related to MS.

CHAPTER 8:

Common Concerns and Detailed FAQs

Can MS be cured? Understanding the current research

Currently, there is no cure for Multiple Sclerosis (MS), but ongoing research is exploring potential therapies that may halt its progression or reverse its effects. Treatments like disease-modifying therapies (DMTs) are designed to reduce the frequency and severity of relapses and slow the progression of disability. Research into stem cell therapy and neuroprotective strategies is also underway, offering hope for future advancements.

Staying informed about new research and clinical trials is essential. Patients can connect with healthcare providers who specialize in MS or join support groups that focus on sharing the latest findings and treatment options. Being proactive in discussions with medical professionals can help patients make informed decisions about their care.

How long can a person live with MS? Life expectancy and quality of life

Life expectancy for individuals with MS can be near normal, especially with advancements in treatment and management strategies. Factors such as the type of MS, the age at diagnosis, and how effectively the disease is managed can influence longevity. Regular medical check-ups and adherence to treatment plans significantly contribute to maintaining a healthy life span.

Quality of life is a vital consideration in MS management. Many individuals with MS lead fulfilling lives, focusing on health, wellness, and support systems. Engaging in regular exercise, nutrition, and mental health care can enhance overall well-being, making it easier to navigate daily challenges.

Can I still have children if I have MS?

Pregnancy and MS

Yes, many individuals with MS can have children, and pregnancy is generally safe for those whose disease is stable. It's important to discuss family planning with a healthcare provider who understands MS, as some medications may need to be adjusted before and during pregnancy. Close monitoring throughout the pregnancy is also essential to manage any potential complications.

Postpartum care is crucial as well, as some women may experience a relapse after childbirth. Ensuring a support system is in place, both emotionally and physically, can help new mothers manage their health while caring for their newborns. Education about MS and its implications can empower individuals during this significant life stage.

Will I need a wheelchair?

Understanding mobility concerns

Mobility concerns vary widely among individuals with MS, and not everyone will require a wheelchair. Some may experience temporary mobility issues, while others might require assistive devices like canes or walkers. Regular physical therapy can enhance strength, balance, and coordination, helping to maintain mobility.

Engaging in adaptive exercises can significantly improve physical abilities and independence. Consulting with healthcare professionals about mobility aids early on can provide individuals with the tools they need to navigate their environment safely and confidently.

How can I manage MS at work or school?

Managing MS in work or school environments involves open communication with supervisors or educators about specific needs and accommodations. Understanding your rights under disability laws can also empower you to request reasonable adjustments, such as flexible hours or modified tasks to support your productivity and well-being.

Creating a supportive network at work or school can further enhance your experience. Utilizing available resources, such as counseling services or peer support groups, can provide valuable emotional and practical assistance, enabling you to thrive in your environment despite the challenges of MS.

Will MS affect my ability to drive?

MS can affect driving ability, primarily if the condition impacts vision, coordination, or cognitive function. It's essential to evaluate your driving skills regularly and consult with your healthcare provider if you notice any changes in your abilities. In some cases, specialized driving assessments can help determine readiness to drive safely.

Many individuals with MS continue to drive safely by managing their symptoms effectively. Staying informed about local regulations regarding driving with a medical condition and considering adaptive driving techniques or vehicles can also help maintain independence on the road.

How do MS affect relationships and intimacy?

MS can introduce challenges in relationships and intimacy due to physical symptoms and emotional changes. Open communication with partners about how MS affects each person can foster understanding and support. It's essential to discuss concerns, desires, and boundaries to maintain a healthy emotional connection.

Engaging in relationship counseling or support groups can provide valuable tools for navigating intimacy issues. Learning adaptive strategies and focusing on emotional intimacy can strengthen relationships, ensuring both partners feel valued and understood despite the challenges posed by MS.

Can lifestyle changes stop MS progression?

While lifestyle changes cannot cure MS, they can significantly impact overall health and potentially slow progression. A balanced diet, regular exercise, stress management, and sufficient sleep can help improve physical and mental well-being. Integrating healthy habits into daily routines empowers individuals to take charge of their health.

Consulting with healthcare providers or nutritionists can help tailor lifestyle changes to individual needs. Engaging in stress-reducing activities, such as yoga or meditation, can also enhance emotional resilience, which is crucial in managing MS effectively.

What should I do during a relapse?

During a relapse, it's vital to prioritize rest and self-care while consulting your healthcare provider for guidance. They may recommend adjusting medications or implementing a specific treatment plan to address the relapse. Keeping a symptom diary can help track changes and patterns, aiding in effective management.

Staying connected with your support network is crucial during this time. Engaging in low-energy activities, like reading or gentle stretching, can help you cope while allowing your body the time it needs to recover. Maintaining communication with friends and family about your needs can foster understanding and support.

Is there a genetic link for MS?

Research indicates that there may be a genetic component to MS, as having a family member with the condition increases the risk. However, MS is a multifactorial disease; meaning environmental factors, lifestyle, and genetics all play a role in its development. Understanding personal and family medical history can provide insights into individual risk factors.

Genetic counseling may be beneficial for individuals concerned about their family history. Staying informed about ongoing research can also provide valuable information about the genetic aspects of MS and potential implications for family planning.

Can stress make MS worse?

Stress can exacerbate MS symptoms and potentially trigger relapses, making stress management an essential aspect of living with the condition. Developing effective coping strategies, such as mindfulness, meditation, or breathing exercises, can help reduce stress levels and improve overall emotional well-being.

Engaging in regular physical activity and seeking support from friends, family, or mental health professionals can also alleviate stress. Building a balanced lifestyle that prioritizes relaxation and self-care can empower individuals to manage their stress more effectively.

Are there alternative therapies for MS treatment?

Alternative therapies can complement traditional MS treatments, although they should not replace medical care. Options such as acupuncture, massage, or herbal supplements may provide relief from certain symptoms. It's essential to discuss any alternative treatments with healthcare providers to ensure they are safe and appropriate.

Exploring lifestyle modifications, such as yoga or nutritional changes, can also enhance well-being. Keeping an open dialogue with healthcare providers about complementary therapies can help integrate these options effectively into an overall treatment plan.

How do I explain MS to children or family members?

When explaining MS to children or family members, it's crucial to use age-appropriate language and reassure them about the condition. Begin by discussing what MS is, focusing on how it affects daily life without overwhelming them with medical jargon. Emphasizing that MS is not contagious and that they can help by being supportive can foster understanding.

Encouraging questions can help address any fears or misconceptions they may have. Sharing personal experiences and feelings about living with MS can also promote empathy and strengthen relationships, allowing loved ones to better support you in your journey.

CHAPTER 9:

Long-Term Management and Lifestyle Modifications

Regular Follow-Up with a Neurologist for Ongoing Care

Regular check-ups with a neurologist are essential for managing Multiple Sclerosis (MS). These appointments allow healthcare providers to monitor disease progression, adjust treatment plans, and address any new symptoms. It's recommended to schedule follow-ups at least every six months, or more frequently if you notice changes in your condition. During these visits, be prepared to discuss your symptoms, medication side effects, and any questions you may have regarding your health.

Additionally, it is helpful to keep a record of any changes or concerns before each appointment. This not only provides your neurologist with detailed information to make informed decisions about your treatment but also ensures that you don't forget to mention important issues during the appointment. Engaging in open communication with your healthcare provider fosters a partnership that can enhance your care and improve your quality of life.

Adapting to Changing Physical and Cognitive Abilities

Living with MS often requires adjusting to changes in physical and cognitive abilities. Understanding that these changes can fluctuate is crucial. Utilize assistive devices, such as canes or walkers, to maintain mobility and enhance independence. Additionally, consider occupational therapy to adapt your home environment, making it more accessible and easier to navigate. This could involve rearranging furniture, installing grab bars, or using adaptive tools for daily tasks.

Cognitive changes may include difficulties with memory, attention, or processing speed. Implementing strategies like using reminders, keeping a structured daily routine, and breaking tasks into smaller steps can be beneficial.

Engaging in cognitive exercises and seeking support from a mental health professional can also aid in coping with these challenges. Building a strong support system with family and friends can provide emotional assistance and practical help.

The Importance of Maintaining a Positive Outlook Despite MS Challenges

A positive outlook plays a vital role in managing the emotional and psychological aspects of MS. Maintaining hope and focusing on the aspects of life you can control—such as your daily activities and self-care—can significantly impact your overall well-being. Engage in activities that bring you joy, whether it's a hobby, spending time with loved ones, or practicing mindfulness techniques like meditation or yoga.

Surrounding yourself with a supportive network can also enhance your mental resilience. Consider joining MS support groups, either in-person or online, where you can share experiences and learn from others facing similar challenges. Celebrating small achievements and setting realistic, short-term goals can foster a sense of accomplishment, keeping you motivated to navigate life with MS positively.

Financial Planning and Managing Long-Term Medical Expenses

Managing the financial aspects of MS requires careful planning and proactive strategies. Begin by assessing your current insurance coverage and understanding what services, treatments, and medications are covered. Contact your insurance provider to clarify details, including out-of-pocket costs, deductibles, and coverage limits. This knowledge will help you budget effectively for ongoing medical expenses.

Consider consulting a financial advisor who specializes in healthcare costs. They can guide you in creating a long-term financial plan that accounts for potential future expenses related to MS, such as additional treatments or assistive devices. Research assistance programs and resources from nonprofit organizations that may help offset costs, including grants and financial aid for medications. Staying organized with records and receipts can also simplify the financial management process.

Staying Up-to-Date with MS Research and New Treatments

Keeping informed about the latest research and treatment options for MS is crucial in managing your condition effectively. Subscribe to reputable medical journals, MS advocacy organizations, and newsletters to receive updates on new studies, clinical trials, and treatment advances. Online platforms and social media can also provide timely information and foster connections with the MS community.

Discuss potential new treatments with your neurologist during appointments. They can help you understand the implications of emerging therapies and whether they might be suitable for your condition. Actively participating in clinical trials may also be an option; it not only contributes to advancing MS research but can provide access to cutting-edge treatments.

Developing a Long-Term Care Plan with Family and Caregivers

Creating a comprehensive long-term care plan is essential for managing MS effectively. Start by having open discussions with family members and caregivers about your needs, preferences, and any potential future challenges. This conversation should encompass medical care, daily living support, and emotional needs, ensuring that everyone involved understands their roles and responsibilities.

Documenting this plan helps ensure clarity and provides a reference for everyone involved. Include details about healthcare preferences, contact information for healthcare providers, and specific tasks for family members, such as transportation to appointments or assistance with daily activities. Regularly revisiting and updating this plan as your condition changes can help maintain its effectiveness.

Managing Medications and Keeping Track of Side Effects

Effective medication management is crucial for MS treatment. Start by creating a medication schedule that outlines when and how to take each prescribed drug. Utilizing a pill organizer or setting alarms on your phone can help you remember doses. Keeping an updated list of medications, including dosages and purposes, will also be beneficial during doctor visits.

Tracking side effects is equally important for effective management. Keep a journal detailing any side effects experienced, along with the date, time, and severity. This information can assist your healthcare provider in adjusting your medication regimen, ensuring optimal efficacy while minimizing adverse effects. Open communication about side effects fosters a collaborative approach to managing your health.

Preventing Secondary Conditions (e.g., Infections, Bone Density Loss)

Preventing secondary conditions is a critical aspect of managing MS. Prioritize a healthy lifestyle, including a balanced diet and regular exercise, to boost your immune system and overall health. Engage in weight-bearing exercises to help maintain bone density, which can be affected by MS-related inactivity or certain medications.

Stay vigilant about infection prevention by practicing good hygiene, including regular hand washing and staying updated on vaccinations. Discuss with your healthcare provider which vaccinations are recommended for your situation. Additionally, monitor any signs of infections or complications early, as prompt treatment can prevent worsening conditions.

Exploring Community Resources and Assistance Programs

Community resources can significantly enhance your quality of life when living with MS. Start by researching local MS organizations, which often offer support groups, educational programs, and resources for those affected by the disease. These organizations can also connect you with local assistance programs that provide financial aid, transportation services, or home modifications.

Consider reaching out to social services or community health organizations to identify additional resources. Many areas have programs specifically designed to assist individuals with disabilities, providing valuable support in various aspects of daily living. Engaging with community resources can foster connections, reduce isolation, and empower you to navigate life with MS more effectively.

Long-Term Exercise and Rehabilitation Plans

Establishing a long-term exercise and rehabilitation plan is vital for maintaining mobility and overall health with MS. Start by consulting with a physical therapist who specializes in neurological conditions. They can design a personalized exercise program that incorporates strength training, flexibility exercises, and aerobic activities suited to your abilities and goals.

Incorporating regular exercise into your routine can enhance physical function and improve mood. Aim for at least 150 minutes of moderate aerobic activity each week, as recommended by health guidelines. Remember to listen to your body and adjust your exercise intensity as needed. Joining exercise classes tailored for individuals with MS can also provide motivation and a sense of community.

Planning for Future Mobility Challenges (Home Modifications, Transportation)

As MS progresses, planning for potential mobility challenges becomes essential. Start by assessing your living environment and identifying areas that may require modifications. This can include installing grab bars in bathrooms, ensuring clear pathways, and considering ramps for easier access. Consulting with an occupational therapist can provide tailored recommendations for creating a more accessible home.

Transportation is another critical aspect to consider. Explore options such as accessible public transport or ride-sharing services that accommodate individuals with mobility issues. If you require a vehicle, research modifications that can make driving easier, such as hand controls or wheelchair lifts. Having a comprehensive mobility plan in place helps ensure independence and safety as your condition evolves.

Keeping a Personal Health Journal to Track Symptoms and Progress

Maintaining a personal health journal is a powerful tool for managing MS. Use it to record daily symptoms, medication schedules, treatment responses, and emotional well-being. Tracking these elements helps identify patterns and triggers, providing valuable insights for discussions with your healthcare provider.

Additionally, noting lifestyle changes, dietary habits, and activities can aid in understanding how they impact your health. Regularly reviewing your journal can help you stay motivated and focused on your wellness journey. Consider incorporating reflective writing, where you express thoughts and feelings, as it can provide emotional relief and clarity.

Staying Motivated and Setting Achievable Goals for Life with MS

Setting achievable goals is key to maintaining motivation while living with MS. Start by identifying specific areas you want to focus on, such as physical fitness, social activities, or personal hobbies. Break larger goals into smaller, manageable steps to avoid feeling overwhelmed. Celebrate small victories along the way to reinforce your progress and boost your confidence.

Engaging in goal-setting with family members or support groups can enhance motivation through shared accountability. Regularly revisit and adjust your goals based on your evolving abilities and circumstances. Staying flexible and open to change helps maintain a positive outlook, allowing you to navigate the challenges of MS with resilience and purpose.

Conclusion

Complementary therapies, such as acupuncture, massage, and yoga, can provide additional relief from MS symptoms and enhance overall well-being. While these therapies do not replace conventional treatments, they can be effective in managing pain, stress, and fatigue when used alongside medical care.

To explore complementary therapies, research local practitioners who specialize in MS or seek recommendations from healthcare providers. It's essential to discuss any complementary approaches with your medical team to ensure they align with your overall treatment plan and do not interfere with any ongoing therapies.

Staying informed about MS and treatment options is vital for effective self-management. Engage with reputable sources of information, such as healthcare professionals, MS organizations, and support groups. Knowledge empowers you to make informed decisions about your care and advocate for your needs.

To enhance your understanding of MS, consider attending educational seminars, reading relevant literature, and connecting with others who share similar experiences. Actively participating in your healthcare decisions fosters a sense of control and confidence in managing your condition.

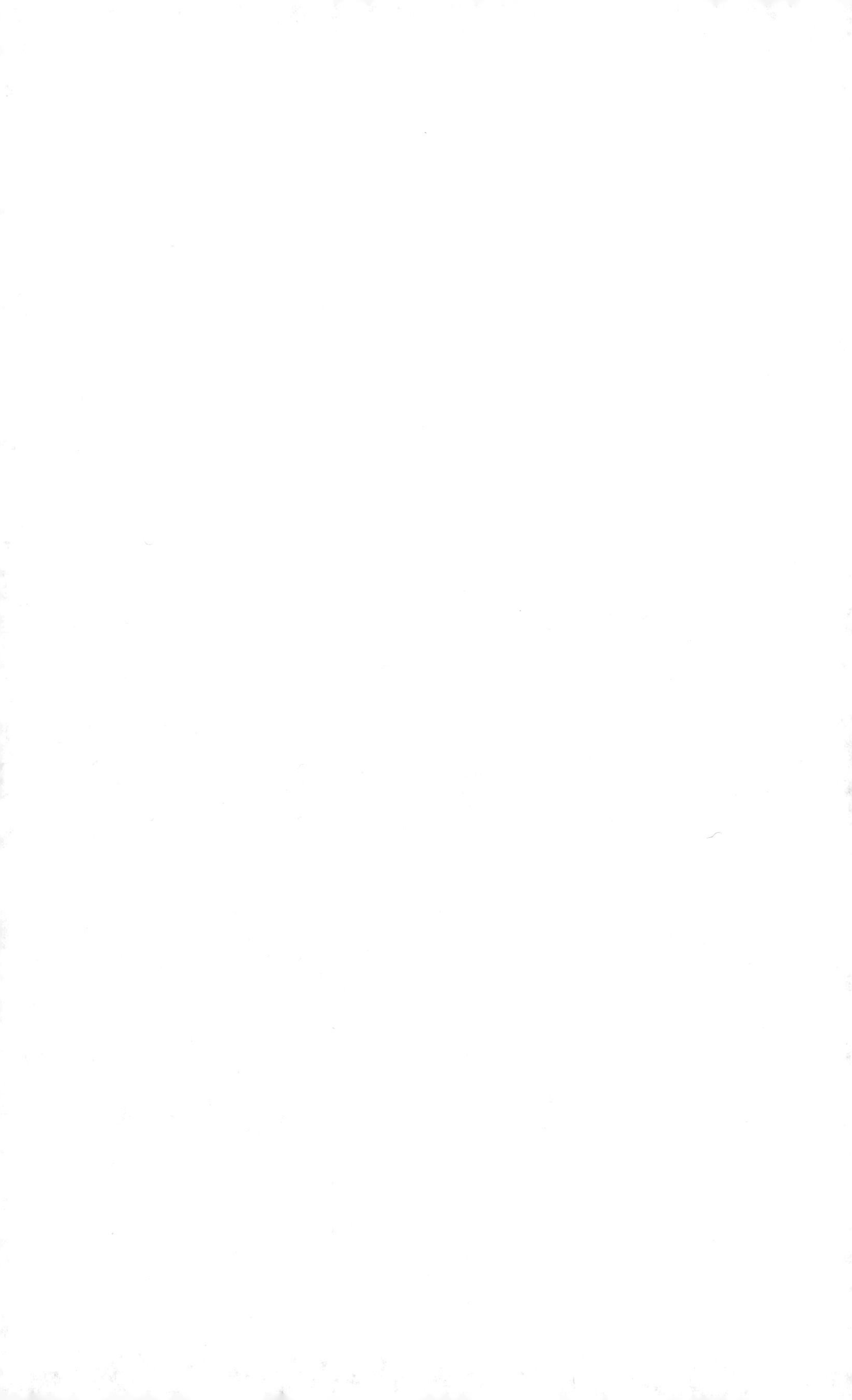

9 798300 381943